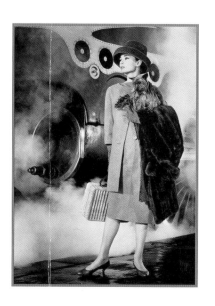

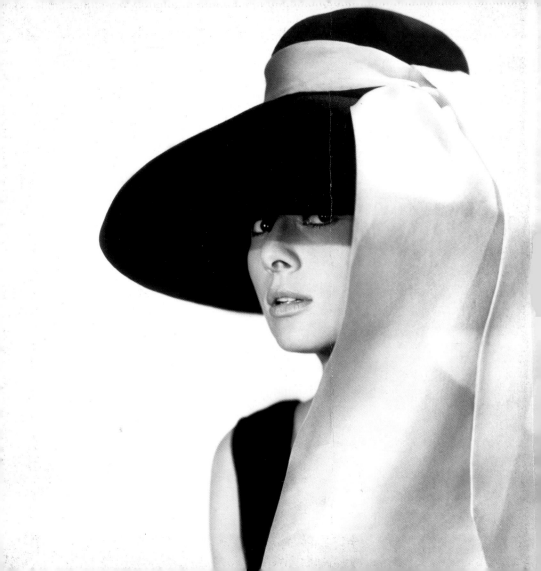

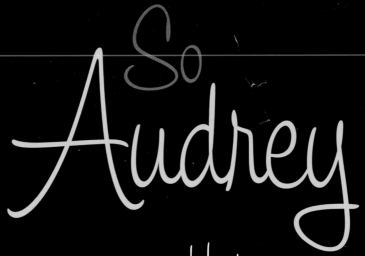

So Audrey

59 Ways to Put a Little *Hepburn* in Your Step

Cindy De La Hoz

RUNNING PRESS
PHILADELPHIA · LONDON

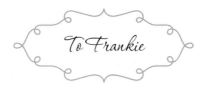

To Frankie

Library of Congress Control Number: 2010926193

ISBN 978-0-7624-4058-0

Designed by Corinda Cook
Photo research by Susan Oyama
Typography: Goudy, Trade Gothic, Brownstone Frames, Ed Script, and Corinthia

Running Press Book Publishers
2300 Chestnut Street
Philadelphia, PA 19103-4371

Visit us on the web!
www.runningpress.com

Audrey Hepburn

excelled like no one else in three distinct areas of her public life—humanitarian, actress, and the absolute epitome of style. The breadth of her charitable work, helping children all over the world through UNICEF, affected millions. In terms of acting, she won dozens of awards and left behind a legacy of great films that still resonate with audiences today. As if that weren't enough, the woman also taught us all how to achieve style in a manner that's posh, polished, and comfortable, to boot. The name "Audrey" has even become a byword for expressing admiration for simple good fashion sense. Her many admirers, who emulate her style, consciously or not, can hope for the thrill of being told on any given day that their look is "so Audrey!"

While Audrey Hepburn's look has become the essence of the term timeless, it was considered daring in her youth. To appreciate the full import of the lessons she taught the world about fashion, you have to remember that Audrey reached the United States from Europe in the early 1950s, an era when Marilyn Monroe was on the rise and popularizing a shapely hourglass figure with her sexy sense of style. Audrey's was the polar opposite of that look. No one had seen anything like her!

Her face was considered, shall we say, problematic. One of Audrey's iconic movies, *Funny Face*, is a tribute to her "quirky" features; the separate parts—huge doe-like eyes, a prominent nose, full brows, slightly off-kilter teeth—all happened to add up to a perfectly charming face. Hollywood accepted that, but confronted with her gamine figure, the natural inclination for studio designers was to help this girl out—pad the hips, pad the bra, cinch the waist to highlight what curves she did have. What they didn't count on was Audrey's polite but firm resistance to the fashion makeover they had in mind.

Audrey may have been small, but she was no pushover. She had taste and innate fashion sense cultivated during her upbringing in Europe. Most importantly, she knew instinctively what looked good on her, and she wasn't about to let anyone make her look silly. At 5'7", Audrey didn't feel the need to add length to her frame with high heels, so she wore flats, or kitten heels, at best. She preferred slim lines to padded clothes, so she wore fitted tops, crisp button-down shirts, and cropped slacks, often in black.

Feeling pressure to conform from Hollywood stylists, Audrey turned to a then fledgling fashion designer in Paris, Hubert de Givenchy. Together, Hepburn and Givenchy revolutionized the world of fashion through their collaboration on her personal wardrobe and on many of her most famous films. The classic *Breakfast at Tiffany's* alone blessed us with the Little Black Dress and helped popularize kitten heels, streaked highlights, oversized

sunglasses, trench coats, the statement necklace—and yes, eating fruit Danish in the most posh
setting possible.

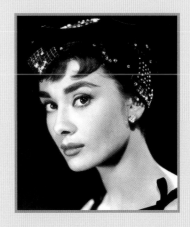

Look at any photo or watch Audrey in *Sabrina*,
Charade, *Funny Face*, *Two for the Road*, or *How
to Steal a Million*, and you'll see why she became
a fashion icon in her own time and for generations
to come. She never thought the attention was
warranted, though. In Audrey's words, "Truly, I've
never been concerned with any public image. It would drive me around the bend if I
worried about the pedestal others have put me on. And also I don't believe it." Audrey's
looks, talent, and good works are not all that make her a fabulous role model for women of
all ages. She also had heart and humility—both wildly attractive traits in a beautiful woman.

This book was inspired by an appreciation for everything about Audrey Hepburn that
makes her a great person to look up to, but as the lady who gave us more timeless wardrobe
pieces than any stylish star, the focus here will be on fashion. What follows are fifty-nine
easy ways that you can put a little Hepburn in your step, and earn that most coveted
of fashion compliments, *"That's so Audrey!"*

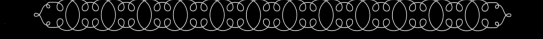

You can never go wrong with a

little black dress.

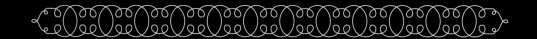

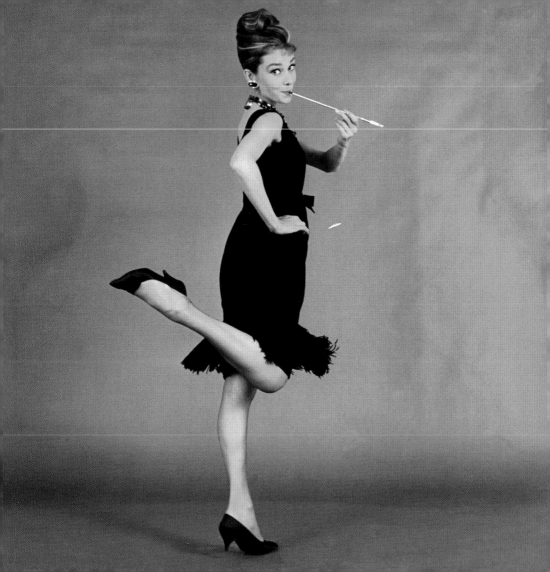

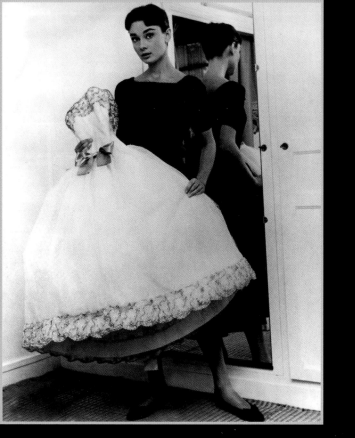

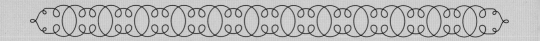

The only competition for the little black dress—

the *little white dress*.

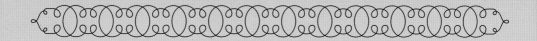

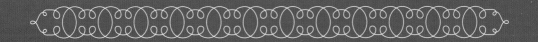

Mix it up with a *splash of color,* to brighten your day.

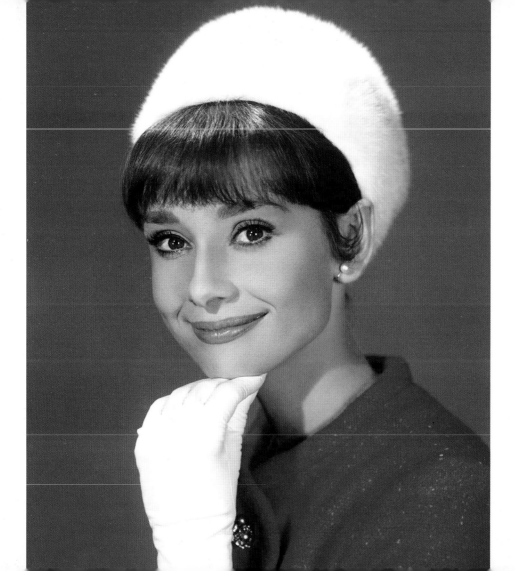

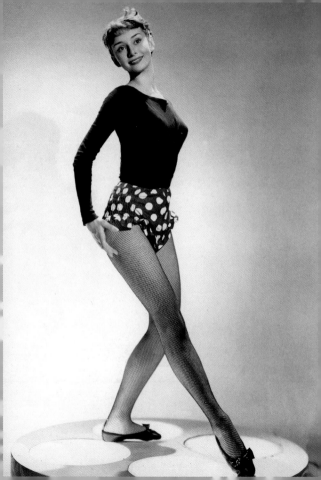

Heels can bring you pain, but a *ballet flat* will never hurt you.

Skip the flip-flops in the summer—

opt for strappy *gladiator sandals.*

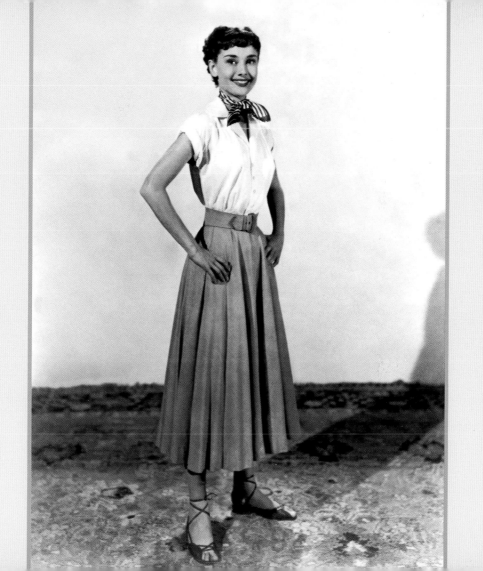

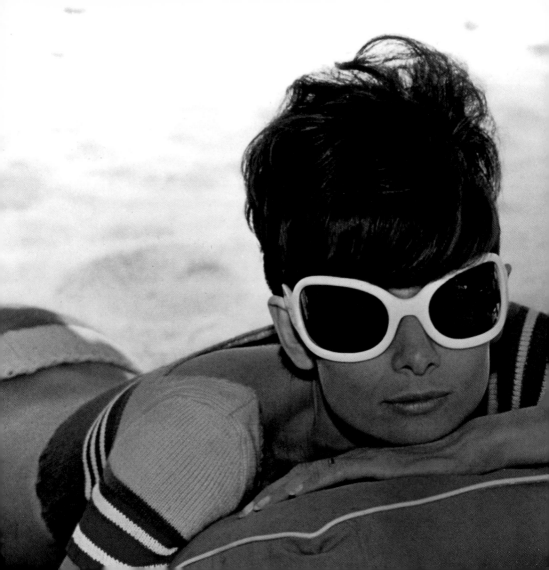

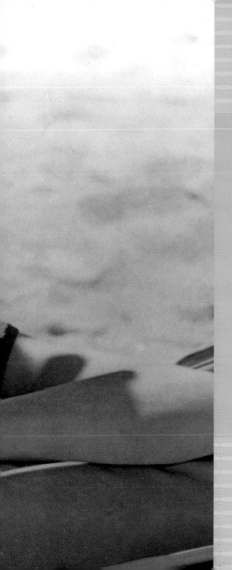

Sunglasses

. . . the larger **the better.**

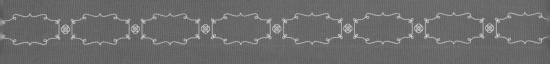

A glorious *sun hat* offers class

—and prevents unslightly squinting.

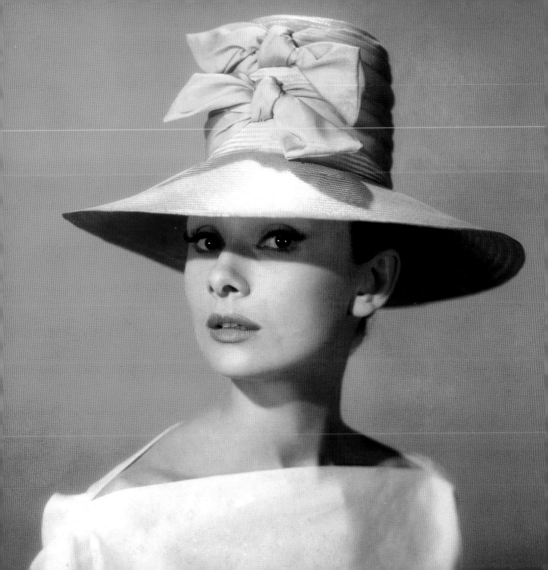

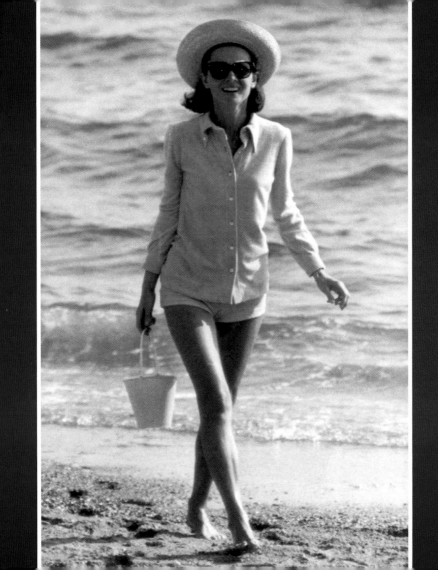

Sometimes *classic menswear* looks better on ladies.

Never underestimate

the importance of *beauty rest.*

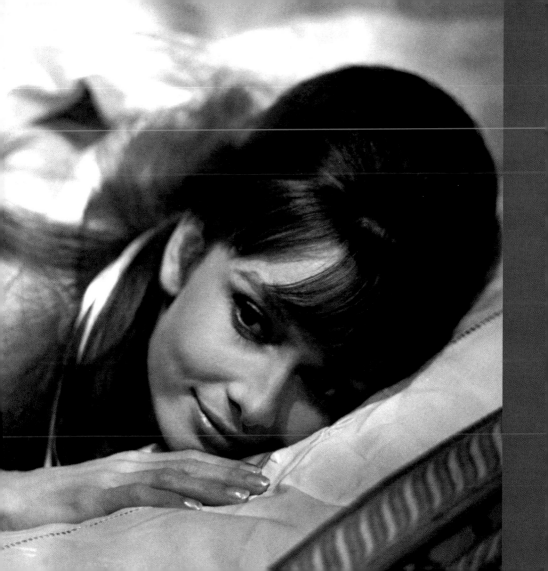

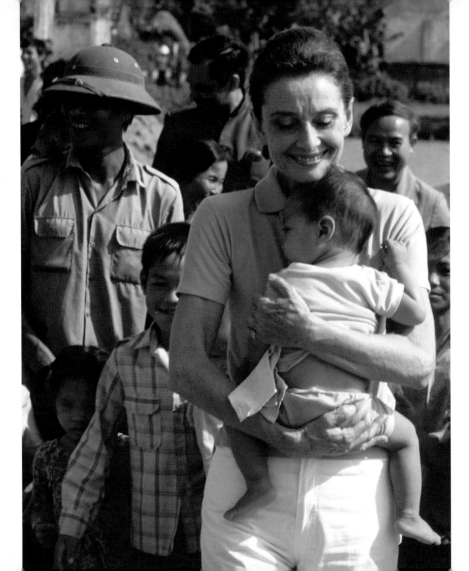

Compassion—

it **wears very well** indeed.

When a late-summer chill hits the air,

always have a *cardigan* on hand.

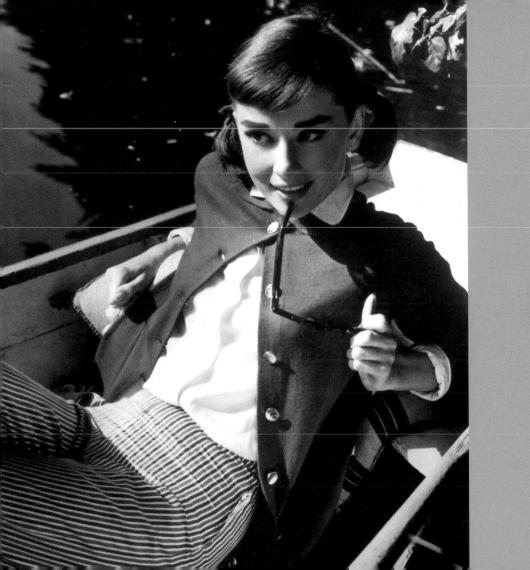

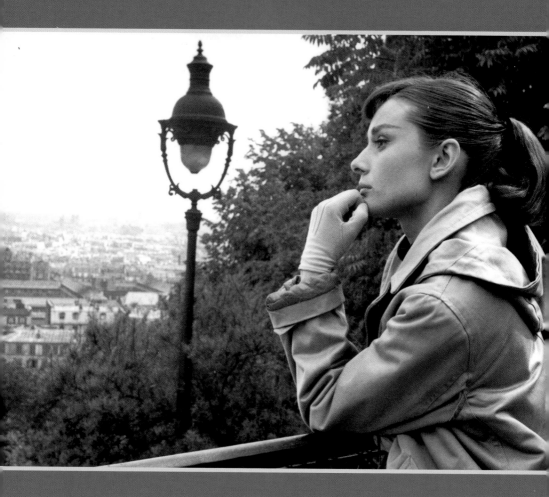

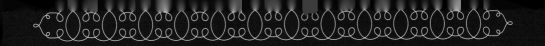

Nothing lends an air of mystery better

than a *classic trench coat.*

Don't question "seasonal pants"

—the effortless style of *white slacks*

is always in fashion.

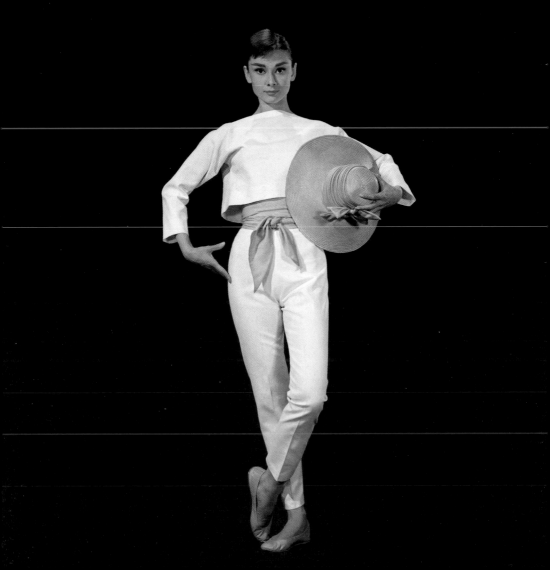

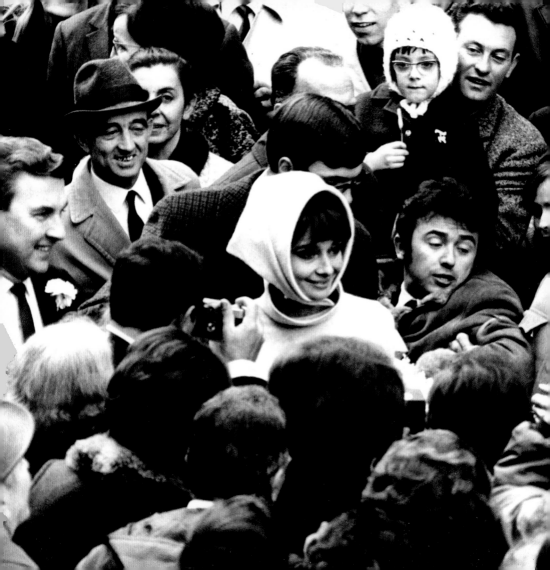

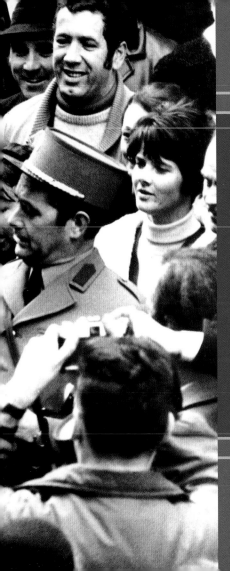

A stylish *headscarf* will always make you stand out in a crowd.

Eyeliner and mascara,

the ultimate dynamic duo.

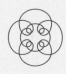

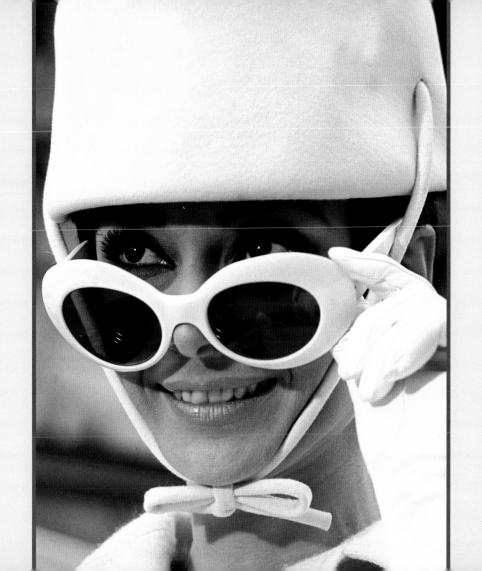

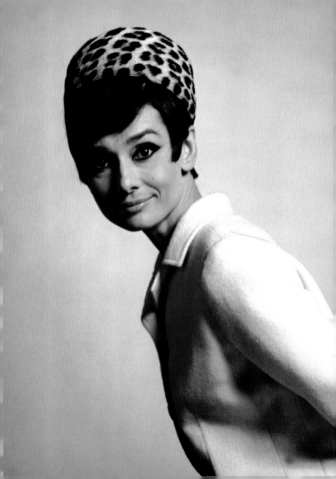

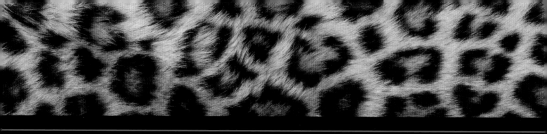

A touch of ultra glamorous *animal print*

goes a long way.

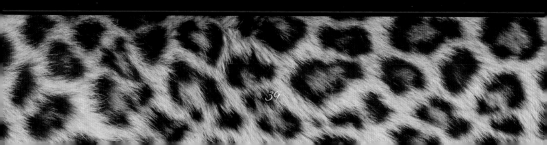

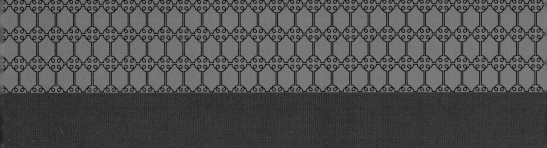

For an unexpected twist,
try a *plunging back* instead of neckline.

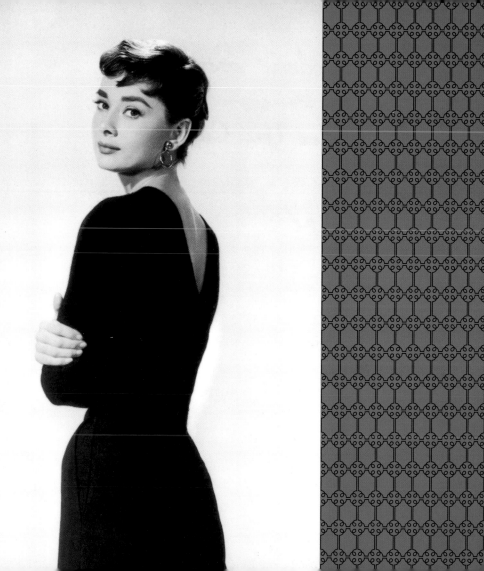

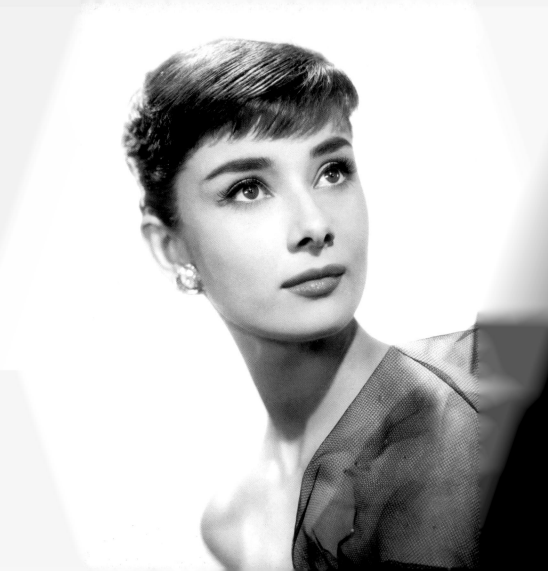

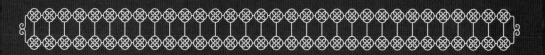

For Audrey it was Givenchy perfume—nothing

lingers in the memory more potently

than a *signature fragrance.*

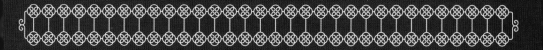

Neatly shaped *full brows* draw attention to the eyes.

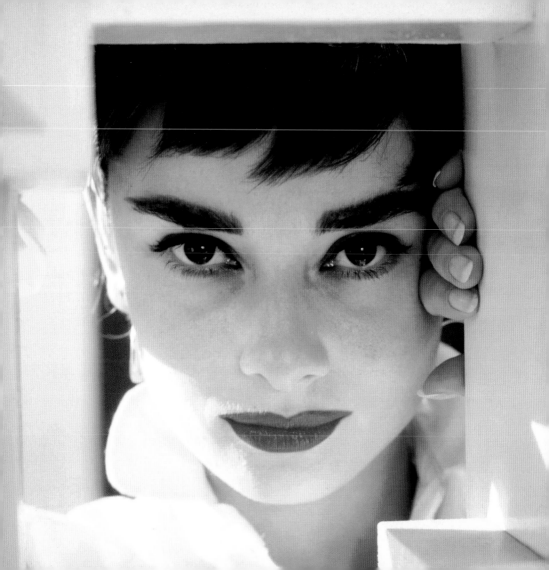

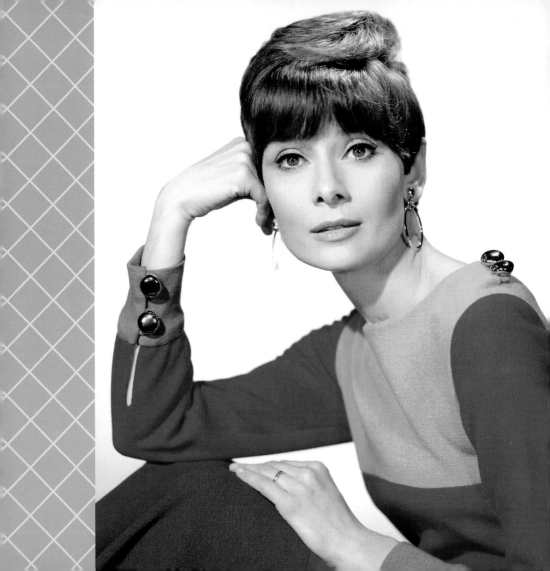

Get into the **bohemian spirit** and

find your ideal *hoop earrings.*

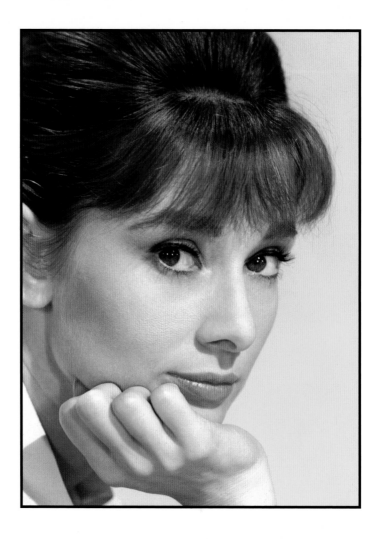

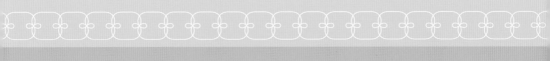

Sideswept, choppy, or straight—

there is a *perfect fringe* for all face shapes.

Don't take fashion too seriously—

let your *sense of humor* shine through.

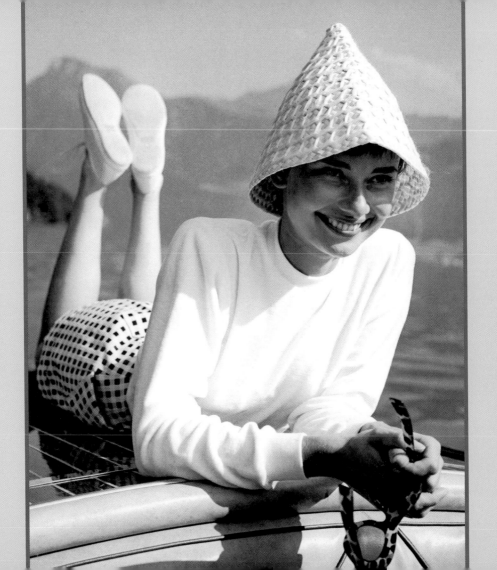

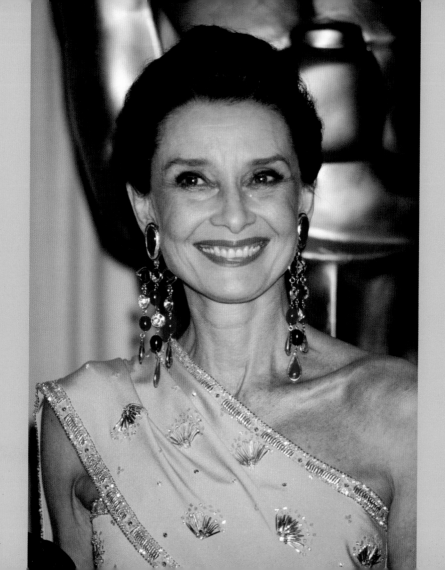

A *one-shoulder dress* equals

instant high fashion.

Perhaps nothing **illuminates** like that

motherly glow.

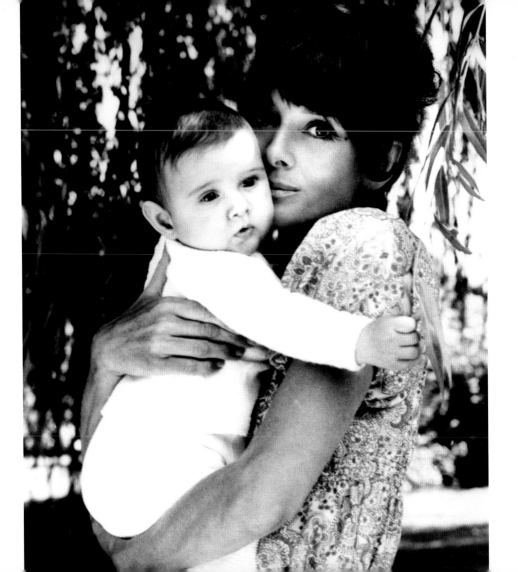

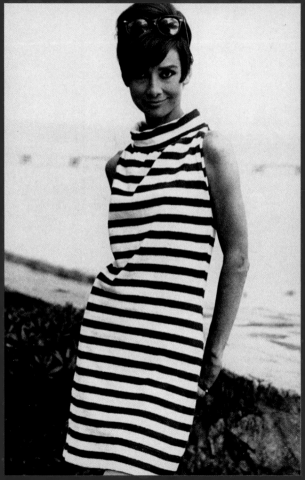

Who says you can't wear

horizontal stripes?

Love the "*funny*
face" in the mirror—

it's the only

one you have.

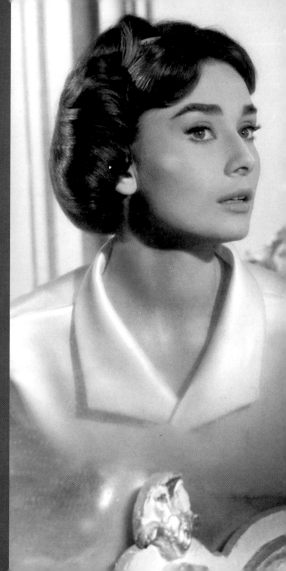

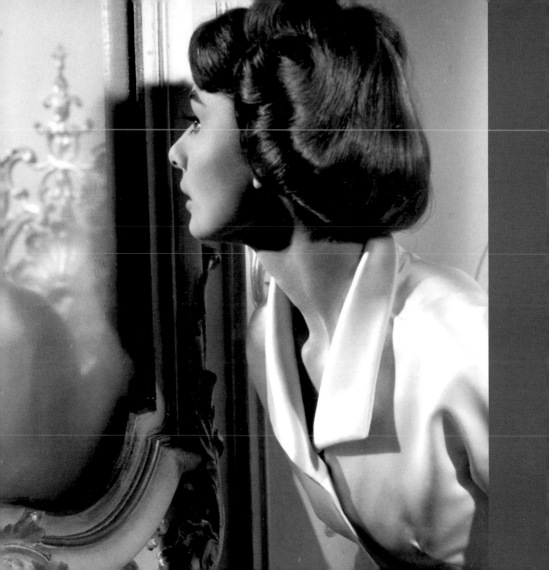

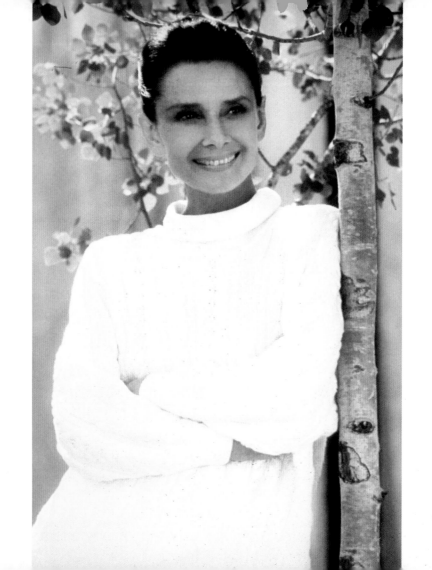

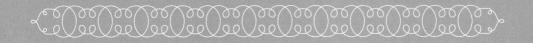

For an **angelic appearance**—

head to toe white.

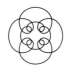

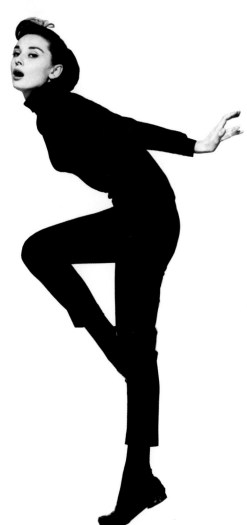

For the essense of the

Left Bank—

head to toe

black.

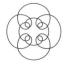

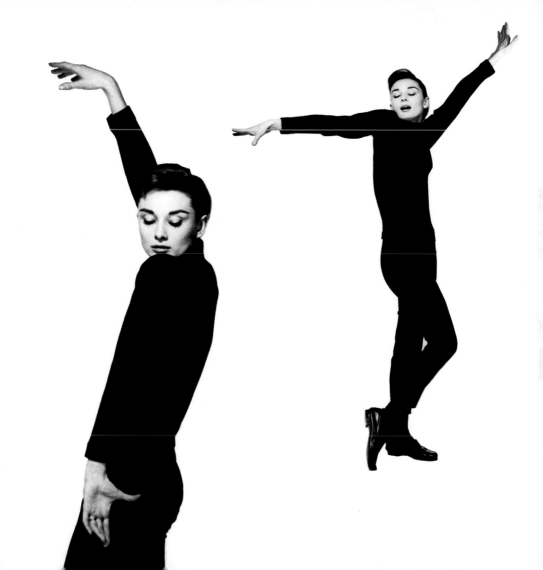

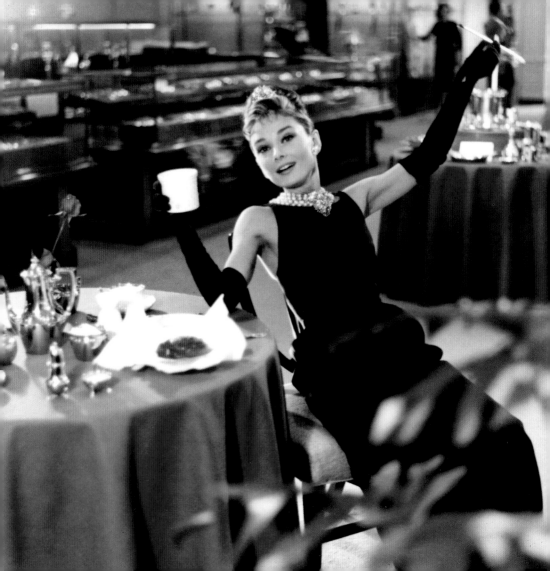

Even a paper cup becomes

elegant when clutched by an

opera glove.

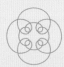

A *smile* is your best accessory—

use it to **spread joy.**

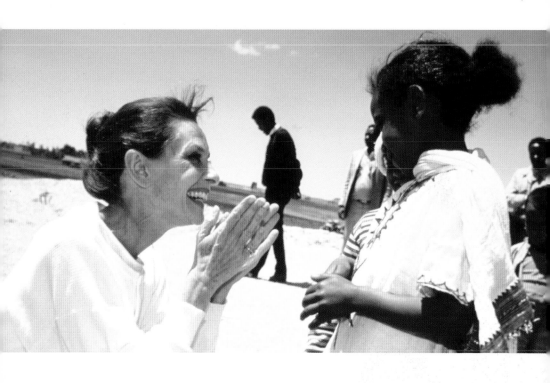

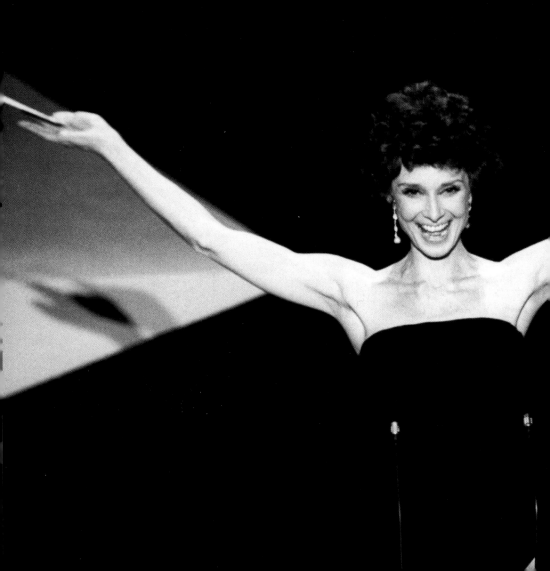

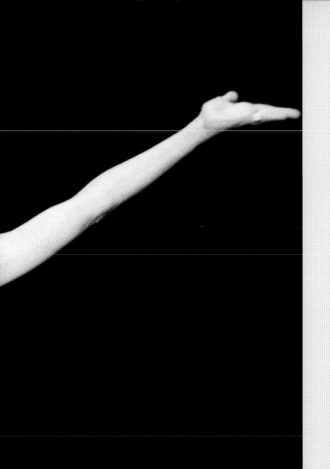

Toned

arms—

always worth a

standing

ovation.

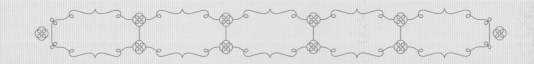

Let a *statement necklace* do the talking.

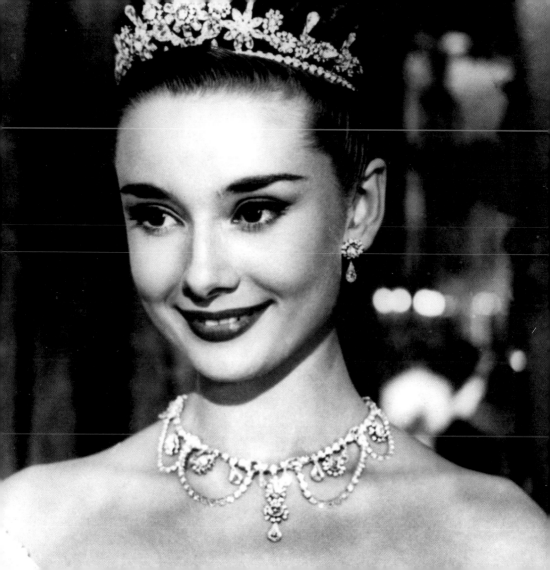

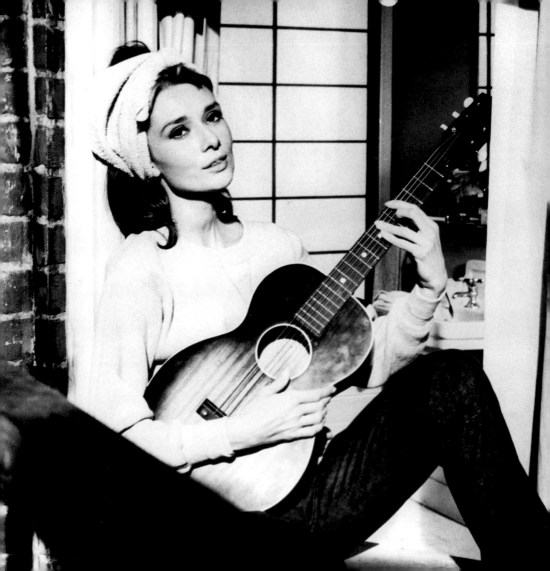

Whether torn for effect, stone-washed,

or dyed indigo, nothing beats a great

pair of *blue jeans*.

A *trusted hairstylist*

is worth their **weight in gold.**

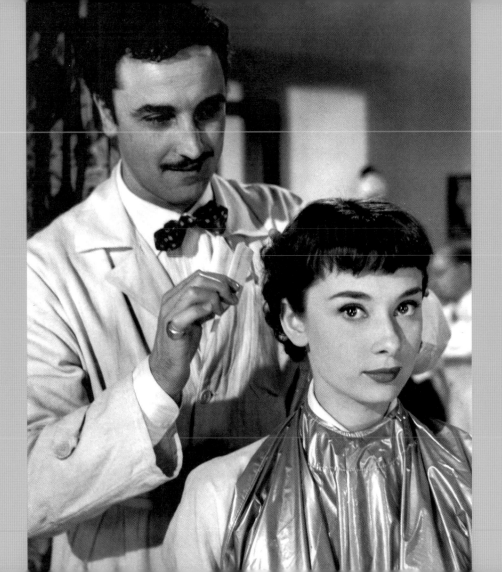

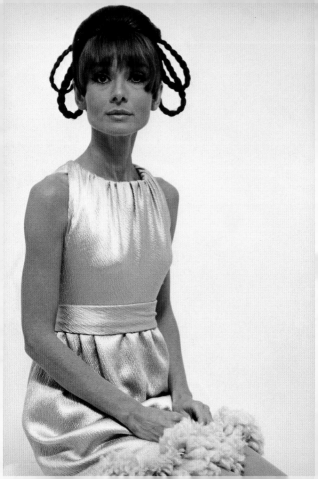

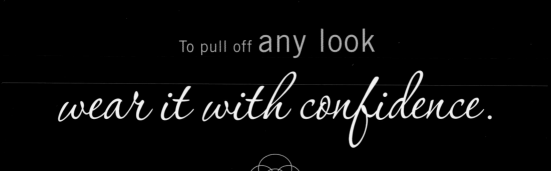

To pull off any look

wear it with confidence.

The *all-purpose scarf,*

tied around the neck, to a belt loop,

or around the head, gives a dash of flair.

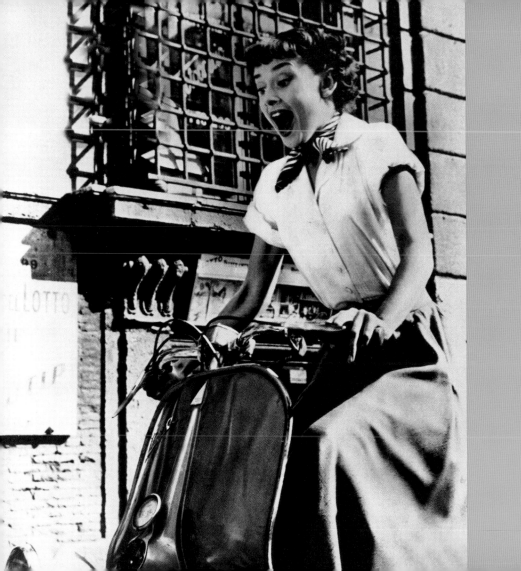

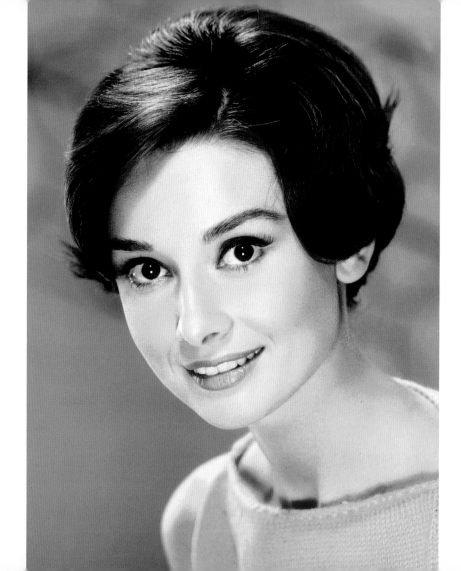

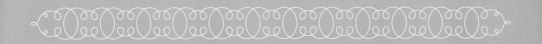

Dramatic eyes and *nude lips—*

a brilliant balancing act.

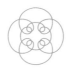

Audrey had a fawn named Ip—

nurture your love of animals

with an *unconventional pet*.

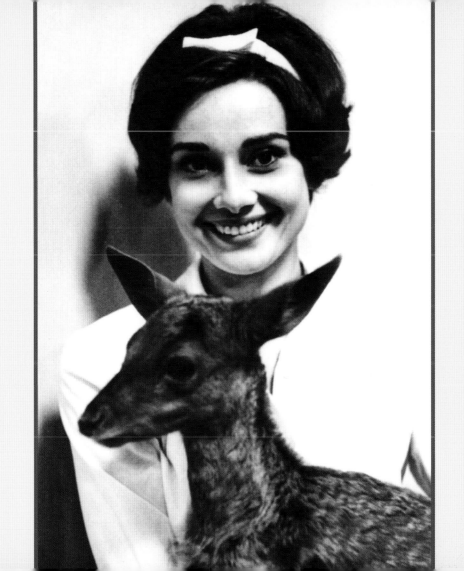

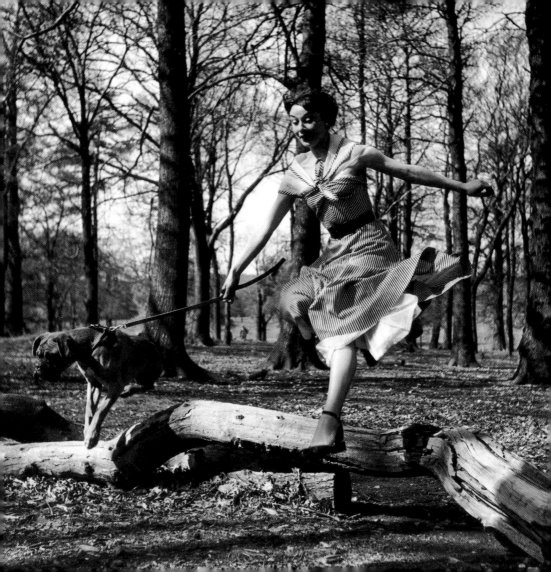

Regular exercise

is more fun with a friend.

A *boat-neck cut* accentuates an elegant collarbone and neck.

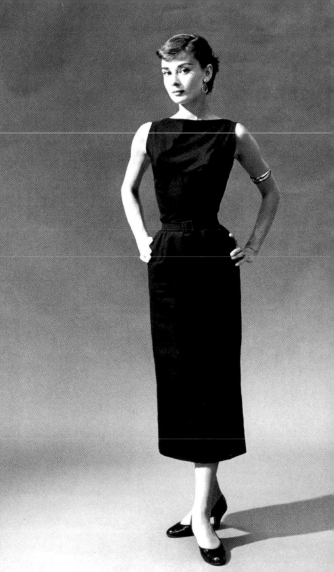

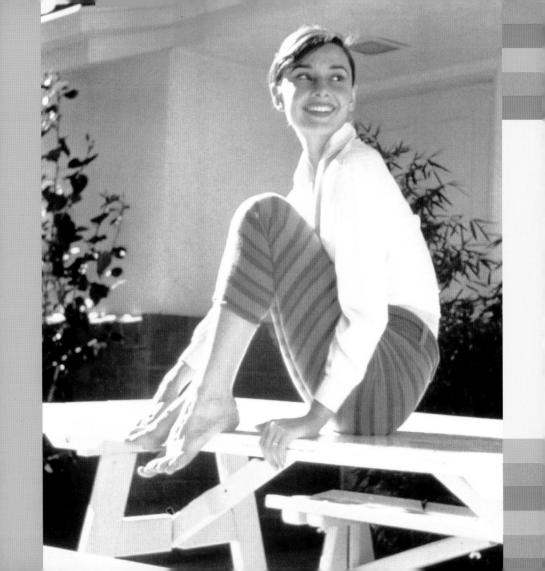

Cropped pants,

in colors or patterned—stock up.

A "mod" fashion staple in the '60s

and **stylish in any era—**

every woman needs a pair of

knee-high boots.

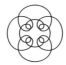

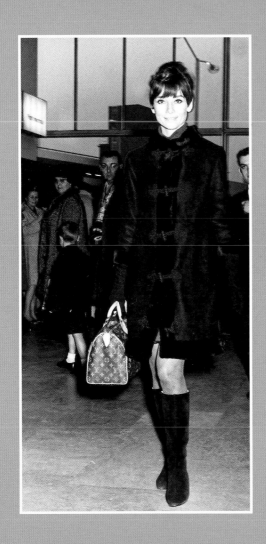

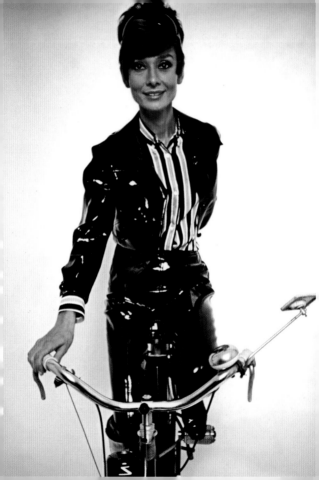

Patent leather—

be it shoes or an entire suit

—always inspires envy.

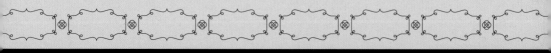

Don't shy away from *unusual*

accessories—

make a statement!

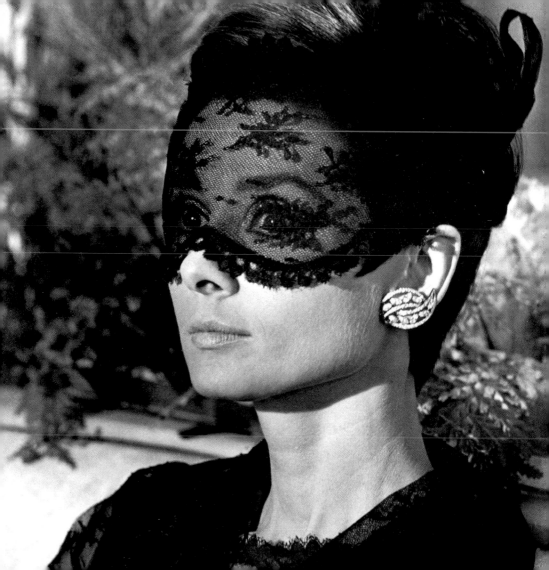

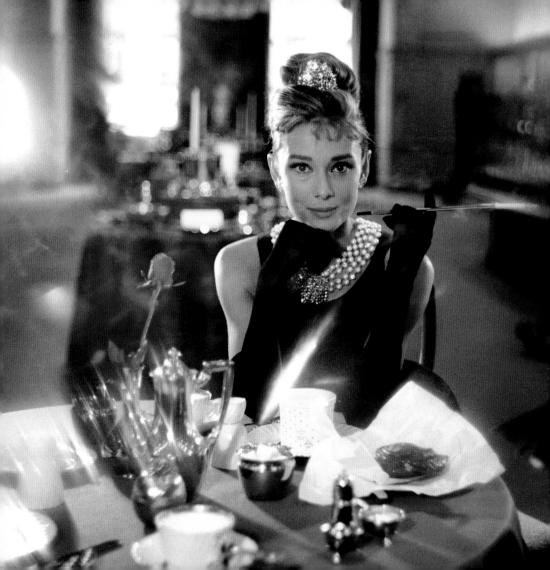

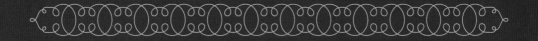

Achieve the **pinnacle of panache**—

study *Breakfast*

at Tiffany's.

A *dose of humility* makes a beautiful woman irresistible.

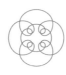

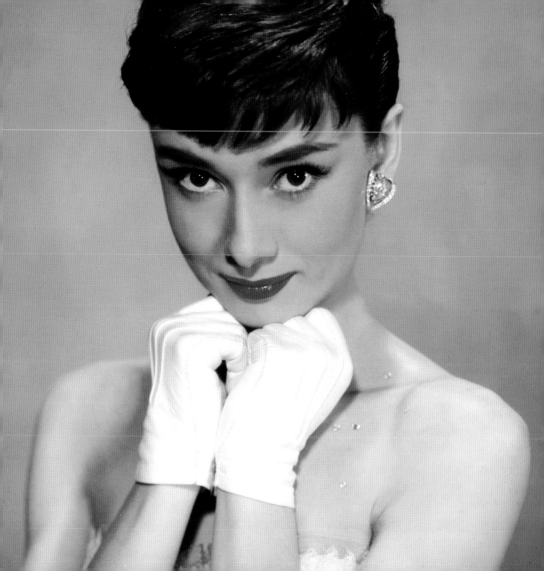

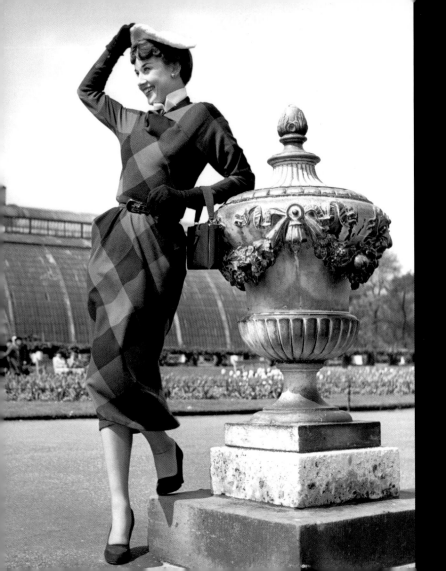

Shoulders back! Any ensemble

can benefit from *good posture.*

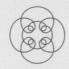

Highlights

are a **streak of genius.**

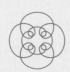

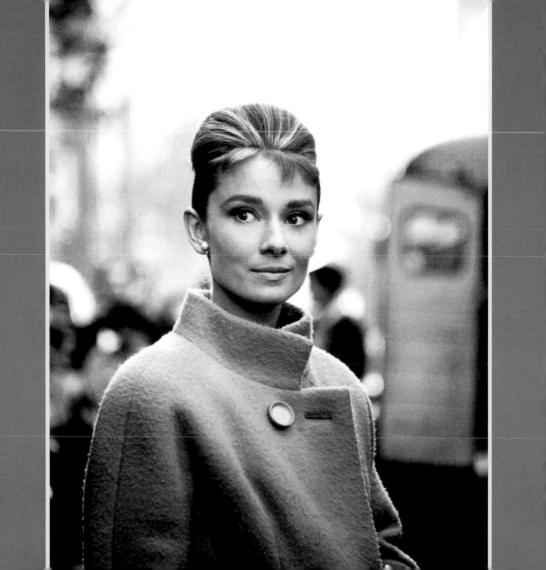

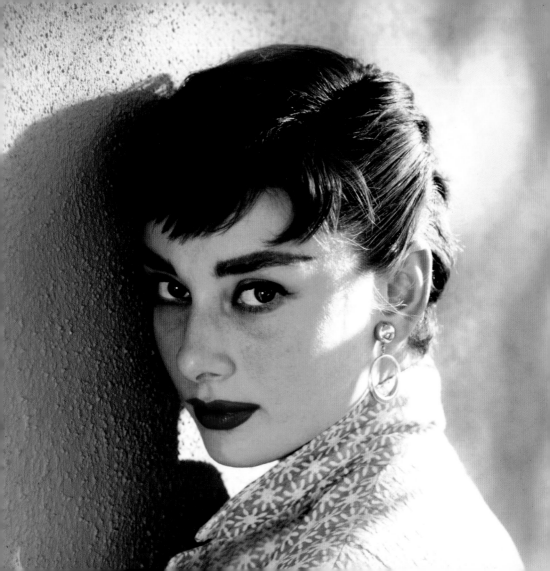

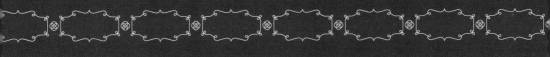

Don't be scared—there is a shade of

red lipstick

for every woman.

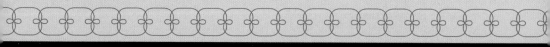

Treat yourself—

an *investment*
handbag is made to last.

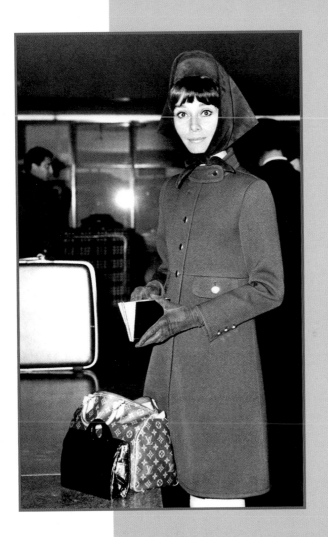

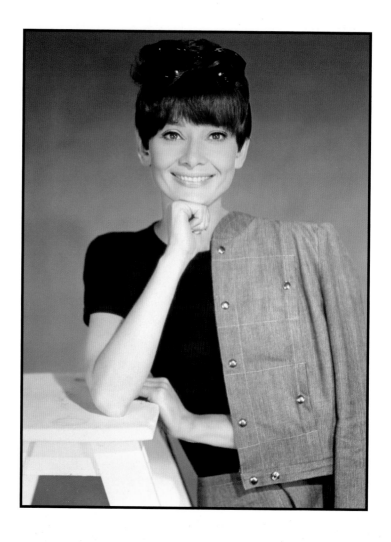

A *denim jacket* is that essential piece to give a lady an edge.

A *healthy diet* is vital,

but when it's your birthday—have your

cake and eat it too.

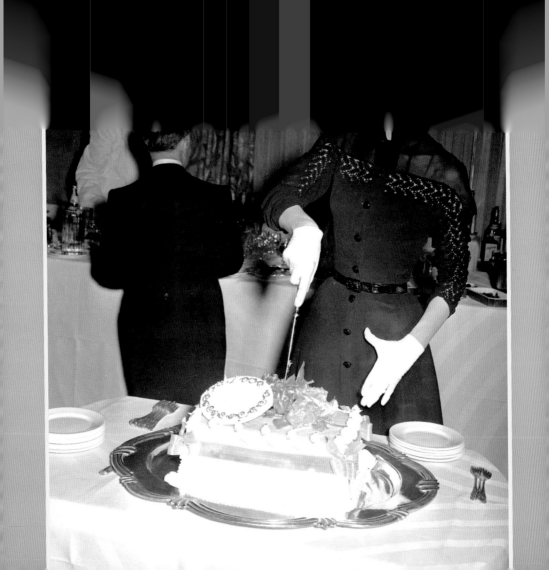

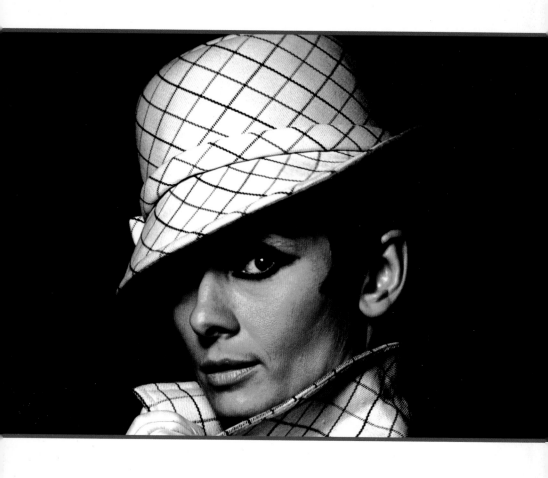

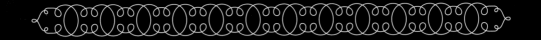

Pop down the brim and wear a *fedora* like you mean it.

Go preppy and playful
with a cute pair of *sailor shorts.*

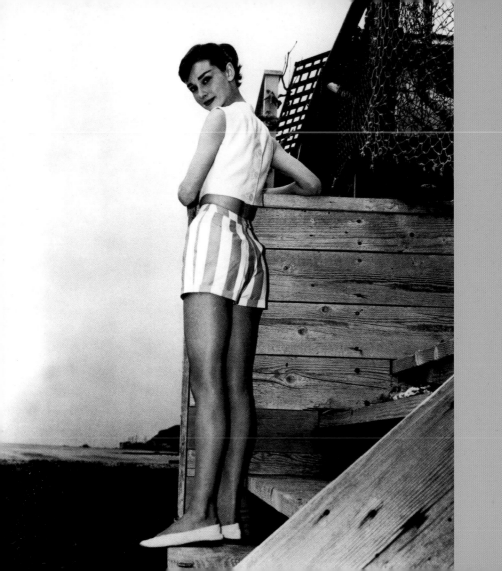

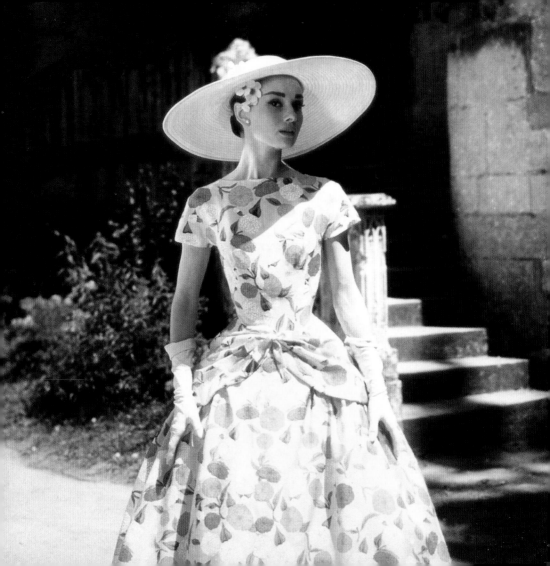

When spring arrives, celebrate with a *floral sun dress.*

Floral arrangements

are clearly **not just for weddings.**

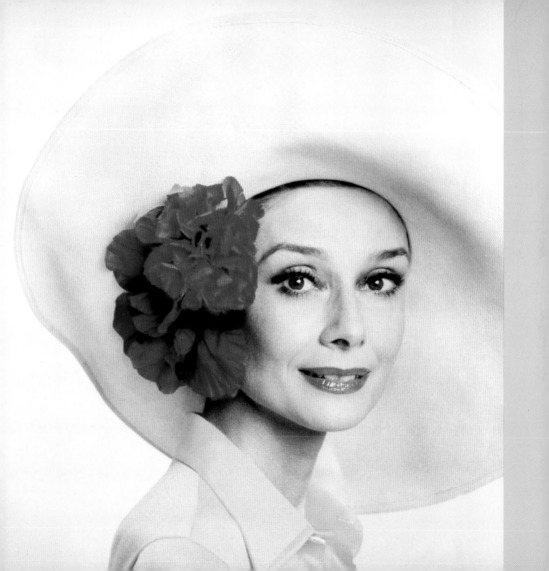

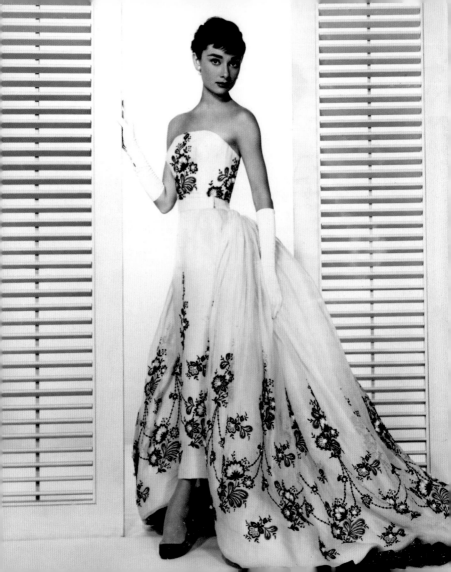

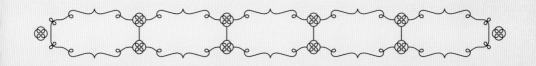

Make a grand entrance

and dazzle the crowd in a *strapless*

evening gown.

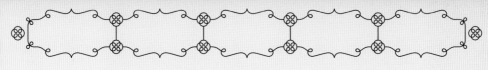

You have a **sense of style**—

pass it on.

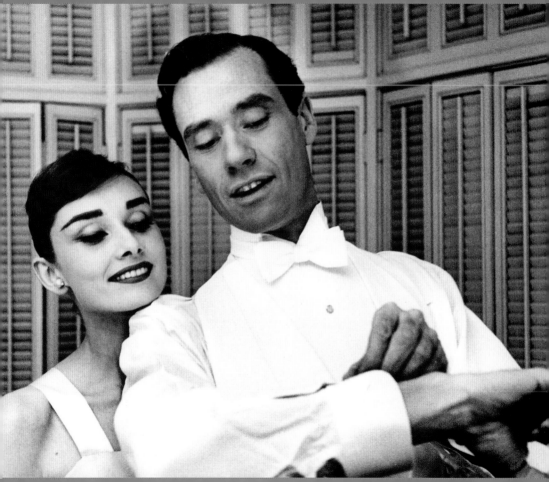

Photography Credits

p. 57: Audrey and son Luca, 1971. ©United Archives GmbH/Alamy

p. 58: Audrey, 1967. Photo By Pierluigi/Rex Features/Courtesy Everett Collection

pp. 60–61: *Love in the Afternoon*, 1957. ©Popperfoto/Getty Images

p. 62: *Always*, 1989. ©Photos 12/Alamy

pp. 64–65: *Funny Face*, 1957. Paramount/The Kobal Collection/Bud Fraker

p. 66: *Breakfast at Tiffany's*, 1961. Paramount/The Kobal Collection/Howell Conant

p. 69: UNICEF Goodwill Ambassador, Ethiopia, March 1988. ©UNICEF/Hulton Archive/Getty Images

pp. 70–71: Academy Awards, 1976. Courtesy CSU Archives/Everett Collection

p. 73: *Roman Holiday*, 1953. ©Photos 12/Alamy

p. 74: *Breakfast at Tiffany's*, 1961. ©Pictorial Press Ltd/Alamy

p. 77: *Roman Holiday*, 1953. ©Photos 12/Alamy

p. 78: *Two for the Road*, 1967. ©20th Century Fox/The Kobal Collection

p. 81: *Roman Holiday*, 1953. ©United Archives GmbH/Alamy

p. 82: Audrey, 1958. The Kobal Collection

p. 85: Audrey, 1959. Courtesy Everett Collection

p. 86: Audrey at Richmond Park, London, May 13, 1950. ©Bert Hardy/Hulton Archive/Getty Images

p. 89: Audrey, 1952. ©George Karger/Pix Inc./Time Life Pictures/Getty Images

p. 90: Audrey, 1956. Courtesy Everett Collection

p. 93: Audrey at Heathrow Airport, London, 1966. Mirror pix/Courtesy Everett Collection

p. 94: *Two for the Road*, 1967. ©20th Century Fox/Courtesy Everett Collection

p. 97: *How to Steal a Million*, 1966. ©20th Century Fox/Courtesy Everett Collection

p. 98: *Breakfast at Tiffany's*, 1961. Courtesy Everett Collection

p. 101: *Sabrina*, 1954. The Kobal Collection

p. 102: Audrey at Kew Gardens, UK, 1950. ©Bert Hardy/Picture Post/Getty Images

p. 105: *Breakfast at Tiffany's*, 1961. Courtesy Everett Collection

p. 106: Audrey, 1954. The Kobal Collection/John Engstead

p. 109: Audrey at airport, Rome, Italy, 1968. Courtesy Everett Collection

p. 110: Audrey, 1967. Courtesy Everett Collection

p. 113: Audrey, 1953. Mirrorpix/Courtesy Everett Collection

p. 114: *Two for the Road*, 1967. Courtesy Everett Collection

p. 117: *Monte Carlo Baby*, 1951. Courtesy Everett Collection

p. 118: *Funny Face*, 1957. Paramount/The Kobal Collection

p. 121: Audrey, 1980s. Courtesy Everett Collection

p. 122: *Sabrina*, 1954. Paramount/The Kobal Collection

p. 125: Audrey and Mel Ferrer. The Kobal Collection/Bill Avery

p. 128: *Breakfast at Tiffany's*, 1961. ©Photos 12/Alamy

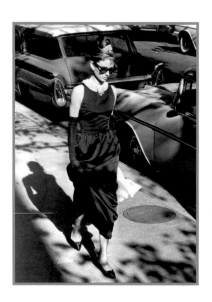

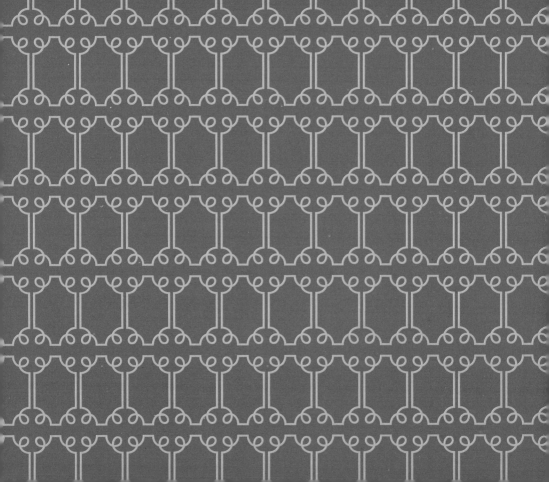